My Journey as a Nurse

My Journey as a Nurse

The Noble Profession

Lynette Shelto-Johnson

Published by Publishing Push Ltd

Copyright 2024 The Lynette Shelto-Johnson book, London, England 2024

First published 2024

English translation 2024

Lynette Shelto-Johnson has asserted her right under the copyright design to be identified as the author of this book. This book is entirely a work of non-fiction.

This book is sold subject to the condition that it shall not by way of trade or otherwise be lent, resold, hired out or otherwise circulated other than that which it is published and without similar condition, including this condition being imposed on the subsequent purchaser.

Limited reference from the internet about Florence Nightingale will be seen in this book.

978-1-80541-488-9 (paperback)
978-1-80541-489-6 (eBook)
978-1-80541-490-2 (hardcover)

Contents

Introduction 1
Who Is Considered a Nurse? 9
    The Nightingale Pledge 10
My Dream of Becoming a Nurse 15
My Pre-Nursing Military Experiences 21
My Practical Nurse Experiences 27
My Life as a Midwife 31
St. Lucia Experience 37
Registered Nurse Accomplished Goal 41
Tapion Hospital, St. Lucia 47
Special Miracles of Life 51
American Experiences 55
Climbing the Career Ladder 59
A Black Person in the Nursing Arena 63
    A Prayer for Nurses and Healthcare Workers .. 64
Reaching Beyond My Career Dreams 67

Giving Up Is Not an Option 71
   Congratulations to My Daughter on
   Her Great Achievements 76
   Graduation of Three Family Members
   on the Same Day: 11 November 2023 76

My Management Work Life 79
   Cultural Day Concert at Work 84
   Birthday Celebrations 85
   Bonfire Night 86
   Unannounced CQC Inspections 87
   15 November 2023 90

Summary 93
   Tips on My Next Book 97

Reasons for Sharing My Stories 99

Acknowledgments 101

Introduction

I learnt that discouraging hours would arise before the rainbow of accomplished goals would appear on the horizon. This was how it was for me when I only had dreams of becoming a nurse at the age of seven years old. I knew somehow I wanted those dreams to become a reality someday. I knew hope was like being in the dark, looking out into the light.

This is how and where my story begins.

As a child growing up, I always admired the nurses' uniform and the way they helped patients on the road to recovery from various illnesses. My mum took me and my other siblings to the hospital for vaccines given by the nurses for all children. Four of these vaccines were for measles, chicken pox, rubella and smallpox. The nurses gave these vaccines to strengthen children's immune systems.

I always wished, prayed and had dreams of becoming a nurse someday. My only fear was needles and having vaccines. I was afraid of needles and even as a grown adult, I am still afraid of them. Thankfully, I do not contract flu quickly and I have never had the flu vaccine due to being afraid of needles. I remembered once, about four to five years ago, I had the flu, and I knew for sure it was the flu. I was sick with aches, pains and a fever.

Regarding the COVID-19 vaccine, I took it against my will, because I could have only kept my job if I accepted the vaccine. The government guidelines mentioned that if workers did not have the COVID-19 vaccines, they would not have been able to continue working by a certain given time. It was indeed a nightmare for me to have an unknown substance in my body. Even the medical team who administered the COVID-19 vaccines did not know what the vaccine ingredients were when I questioned them.

My zeal for becoming a nurse enhanced more when one of my younger sisters died in the same bed next to me. I was about seven years old, and she was about five years old.

Looking back over those years and reminiscing, I remember and have the belief that the nurses overlooked us as children who did not need medical attention. My sister and I did not appear to be sick from the food poisoning, as I remember we were the only two people from the family who were able to move around. If I were a nurse back then, I would have also assumed that my sister was fine and did not need monitoring for food poisoning. Looking back through the years, I faintly remember that I felt nauseated, but

INTRODUCTION

I still was happy to walk the hospital floor to visit my other siblings and mum who were extremely ill from the food poisoning.

That was a dreadful nightmare my family and I encountered. It was a great lesson learnt for us too. This profound and sad story has motivated me to be the best version of a nurse. I have learnt that things are not always as they seem. Also, as the saying goes, do not judge a book by its cover. I know in the medical field there is a triage system, but it is also a promising idea to check all patients in the hospital or if they are at home. There are patients who are unable to express their true feelings about their illnesses.

When my sister died, I vowed to be one of the best nurses to serve humanity and I kept that promise. This I am thankful to God for, and I am thankful for the nurse who I have become today.

The interesting contents of this book will inspire and motivate young people not to give up on their dreams, especially those who have dreams of becoming a nurse someday. After reading this amazing book, you will remember that giving up should not be an option at any point in time. Resilience, motivation and willpower should be applied to avoid negative feelings such as frustration and depression. Especially feelings of discouragement.

Once there is life, there is hope for reaching one's dreams. Rain does not fall forever, and storm clouds always eventually pass over. Sometimes in my dark days, I learnt that doing the things I love helped me to overcome the negative feelings that would bring on unhappiness. I love when the clouds go away and the sunlight shines through. It is a whole brand new feeling of joy. This is how I think about rainy days and cloudy days. I always believe the rain will stop and the sun will eventually shine.

My cousin Vidal once said that you can only shoot an arrow by pulling it backwards first. Sometimes when life is dragging us back with difficulties, it means that it will launch us into something great. This amazing and inspiring book outlines the struggles during my journey to a successful nursing career. With prayer, trust in God and challenging work, I reached success. The good Lord, my families, friends and mentors were there along the way to give me the necessary support and guidance. I also learnt that when we help others, we are also helping ourselves.

Through it all, I must say that I have achieved my career dreams and I thank God.

My passion to become a good nurse and to help save the lives of people was enhanced because the nurses' and doctors' assumptions about my sister were wrong. They thought my sister and I were not so ill from the food poisoning. The medical team's assumption was wrong because my sister died because of ineffective investigation and limited observation.

INTRODUCTION

I am older and wiser now, so my reflection on this historic nightmare has improved my knowledge of becoming a nurse with excellent investigation and observation skills.

My father on occasion told me that I would become a nurse someday and his thoughts were correct. He used to say things that materialised, so people used to call him a special gifted man.

It was a promise I kept, and despite challenges, I am a registered nurse and midwife, and now a registered care home nurse manager, care home trainer and part-time writer.

I delivered babies in my younger days and one of my deliveries was my niece Mellissa. I can never forget when I delivered Mellissa; she was not breathing when she came into this world. I was determined by the help of God to practise the midwifery skills I had to make Mellissa cry, to promote an effective airway. Finally, Mellissa began to cry. Her cry was not loud, so I asked another midwife to take Mellissa and complete the airway suctioning to open Mellissa's airways more effectively. This gave me more time to deal with my sister Jennifer, as the placenta was still inside the uterine cavity. The other midwife finally returned with Mellissa giving a loud cry. I was so happy. My sister Jennifer was also incredibly happy too, as she did not get the chance to hold Mellissa right away at birth. This was because at birth Mellissa needed urgent attention. Jennifer was happy to hold Mellissa and she was overjoyed. As a grown adult now, Mellissa sometimes jokes that I beat her as soon as she was born. This is because I had to give her back taps to help open her lungs.

I decided to share this story in the introduction of my book because it taught me that giving up should not be an option when trying to be successful at anything.

Delivering so many babies, I knew that one day that I would need a child or children of my own. Speaking about delivering babies, I remember on night duties, babies used to be born more often than during the day. Sometimes the night duties were tiring and exhausting but once the babies were ready to come into the world, tired or not, I had to get the job done. It was an amazing feeling when the babies cried at birth. The smiles on the mothers' faces were happy, heartwarming and priceless. When a baby comes into this world, I see that as a miracle and an act of God's divine intervention and creation. They are usually priceless moments that lead into minutes, hours, weeks, months and years. It is always a wonderful feeling when a child is born.

I was so entangled with my nursing career for years, with my assistant nurse programme, my midwifery programme and much more. When I got married at thirty-two, I had three miscarriages. The gynaecologist

INTRODUCTION

told me I waited too long to have a child. He also told me it could be hormonal changes causing an unfavourable uterine environment, which was causing the miscarriages. I prayed about it as I was not ready to give up on having a child based on one gynaecologist's ideas and assumptions.

One year later my daughter Crystal was born by the grace and mercies of God. The gynaecologist who said I may not have children called my daughter a wanted baby during my pregnancy. After I had a caesarean section for the birth of my daughter, he called my daughter a miracle baby. I knew then that nothing is impossible with God. I was overjoyed and gave praise and thanks to Almighty God.

I chose to name my daughter Crystal. This is a girl's name of Greek origin. Crystal symbolises something clear or precious. I pray that God will grant her a clear path with remarkable success in life and that Crystal will be grateful to God for protecting her during my pregnancy and during her life so far.

This is another interesting story of my life that I thought I should add to the introduction of my book, as it was a great miracle in my life story of how God can turn impossibility into possibilities. This was a wonderful miracle during my nursing career journey when God blessed me with my beautiful daughter.

This book will not only captivate the hearts of aspiring nurses and regulated registered nurses, but it will also inspire anyone who reads it. Its contents are motivating, inspiring, emotional, uplifting and encouraging.

I focused a great deal on why people should never give up on their dreams. My book will also help you with personal brokenness and personal revival in any job aspects, but mostly in the nursing arena.

The introduction will also make you want to dive deeper and deeper into the various chapters. I hope you enjoy reading the rolling contents of this book. Miracles sometimes happen when we least expect them. Sit back, relax and enjoy your read.

Who Is Considered a Nurse?

First, a nurse needs to be qualified before they can start the full responsibilities of a nurse. This is someone who takes care of the patient after the registration process.

A nurse is someone who conducts a noble, fruitful, medical, amazing and divine profession. God created this profession to aid in the initiative-taking process, investigatory phrase, treatment plan, healing process and recovery process of someone who is physically, emotionally and mentally unwell. Others may have many other meanings for who a nurse is.

Florence Nightingale was known as "the Lady with the Lamp". Her stories have inspired me and millions of other nurses around the world. She was born in the eighteenth century in 1820 and she died in 1910. Florence was a trainer and manager for nurses during the Crimean War. This amazing nurse cared for soldiers during the war and her life has left great lessons for all nurses.

The Nightingale Pledge

I solemnly pledge myself before God and in the presence of this assembly to pass my life in purity and to practise my profession faithfully.

I will abstain from whatever is harmful and mischievous and will not take or knowingly administer any harmful drug.

I will do all in my power to maintain and elevate the standard of my profession and will hold in confidence all personal matters committed to my keeping and all family affairs coming to my knowledge in the practice of my calling.

With loyalty will I aid the physician in his work, and as a missioner of health, I will dedicate myself to devoted service for human welfare.

This career and the people who are in this career like me used to be highly respected years ago. I cannot say that this is the same case today. People verbally abuse nurses today. Sometimes even physically abuse them. This is a sad thing.

Centuries ago, anyone who had the knowledge to help in the medical field used to deal with the sick. Despite there being legal requirements today to care for the sick, there are still people who help to care for the sick without a nursing certificate. The elderly people used to care for the sick mostly at home. The hospitals never had so many patients like they do today. People used to visit the hospitals only for real emergencies, as the local communities' elderly were skilled enough to care for the sick. There were also community nurses who used to visit the small communities and give help where needed. Anyone who thought they were capable used to be able to give first aid help in ancient days. This was a significant help for the hospitals.

My mum never went to a nursing school, but she too used to help look after us if we had a fever. She was exceptionally good at fever management and she used to help outsiders too. This she used to do free of charge. My mum was an exceedingly kind and helpful person. The same was with my dad. He was very gifted at healing people with bush medicine. I am not sure how he knew which bush helped with which condition, but it was amazing how it worked. In Guyana there is a bush by the name of fever grass. The Guyanese boil it and make tea. It has fever reducing properties they believe. My mum and dad used to give us fever grass tea. As far as I can remember, it worked. My mum boiled senna leaves every Sunday and gave the tea to my siblings and me. She believed it would keep away constipation, which it did.

My mum and dad were doctors and nurses in their own little way, and this has helped us a great deal. It kept us from too many hospital visits. My mum only took us to the hospital when it was obviously necessary.

My mum was very skilled in fever and cold management. If we had a fever, cold and cough, she used to make her own cough medicine which used to help with the coughing. These home remedies prevented frequent hospitals visits.

To be a registered nurse today, a trained nurse legally has to train in a nursing school or university for three or four years depending on the country's policy. Those years of training will cover the various aspects of nursing which will equip the nurse to be able to care for the sick effectively. After those years of training, there will be a graduation where the nurses will receive their certificates.

After the graduation and the giving of certificates, the nurse, by law, is required to apply for the nursing registration before they can work as a registered nurse.

This is the process in St. Lucia where I worked for fifteen years as a nurse, and it is also the same process in Guyana where I was born.

Induction is legally necessary for any first job the nurse will undertake before being able to work alone without supervision. The unit manager will need to conduct the supervision to make sure the registered nurse is ready to perform duties alone on the unit. This is vital to ensure the safety of all the patients.

WHO IS CONSIDERED A NURSE?

There are various categories of nurses. Nurses complete different types of nursing programmes such as programmes to be a licensed practical nurse, a registered nurse or a mental health nurse. After years of experience and excellent work, nurses receive promotions to ward supervisors, ward sisters or ward matrons. There are nurses who have branched off to becoming doctors, physiotherapists, pharmacists and so much more. Being a nurse calls for patience, motivation, willpower, determination, love, strength, resilience and dedication. It is not an easy job, but a nurse needs to love the nursing profession before they can be a good or excellent nurse.

All nurses should aim for professional excellence which will help them to promote effective nursing care, which should be holistic and person-centred. It should be rewarding and fulfilling. For so many, discouraging hours will arise before the rainbow of accomplished goals. This is why nurses need motivation and encouragement daily. Excellent teamwork and a wonderful team spirit should be encouraged as this enhances effective work.

Nursing in the ancient days had its advantages and disadvantages. Likewise, today, there are so many advanced technologies which are in use to confirm a diagnosis quickly.

Nurses and carers do not have to physically lift a patient anymore, like we did in the days of old. In today's society, nurses and carers have all the various moving and handling equipment, such as the full body hoist, ceiling hoist, standing hoist and Zimmer frame.

This lifting and moving equipment has reduced a number of back injuries for nurses and care workers. It has also reduced falls for the patients. This advanced equipment has really brought about a speedy action plan for moving and handling issues.

Nurses were known for wearing white uniforms. Nurses used to also wear blue and white striped uniforms. Today, nurses wear an assortment of coloured uniforms. It depends on the hospitals' or various medical institutions' uniform policy. I used to enjoy wearing the white nurses' uniform, but I fell in love with the new system of not wearing white uniforms too.

My Dream of Becoming a Nurse

As a child growing up, I always used to love watching the nurses wearing their lovely white uniforms or blue and white striped uniforms. It used to look so beautiful with the white head cap. I always used to wish that one day I would be able to wear the same nurses' uniform when I grew up. I believe at that age of five or six, I was more captivated by the look of the uniform and not actually being a nurse. As I grew up, at the age of seven, wanting to become a nurse started to register in my mind. When my mum took me to the hospital for treatment or vaccines, I used to watch how the nurses completed their work. I began to get interested in the way the nurses conducted their work.

One thing I knew for sure was that I was afraid of needles, and I am still afraid even now. I will never overcome the fact that I am afraid of needles. Even though I am afraid of needles, I am very skilled when it comes to administering injections to a patient. Yes,

I know it sounds strange that I don't like needles and injections, but I give injections to patients.

When I was seven years old, my entire family got food poisoning and we were all hospitalised. My mum was pregnant, and she was the worst one who was sick out of the family. My sister, who was in the same cot with me, did not appear to be sick as she was playing. Unfortunately, the poison took effect on her, and she passed away beside me in the same bed. It was emotionally disturbing to see the nurses taking her away. I remember saying to the nurses not to take my sister away. Looking back now, I realise that once someone has food poisoning, the nurses should check that person whether they are sick or not. Due to that fateful day, I made an oath to myself to be a nurse and help save people's lives by the grace of God.

And that was an oath I carried through with and I kept that promise I made.

Helping people if they had a cut and pretending to be a nurse in my childhood days was something I enjoyed doing.

During my school days, I used to focus on subjects such as biology and other subjects that would help me to pursue my dreams of becoming a nurse. I used to ask the nurses questions about nursing anytime I visited the hospitals.

After completing my secondary school days, I investigated how to get into nursing school.

I migrated from Matthew's Ridge to Georgetown in Guyana in January 1979, following the Jonestown Massacre in November 1978 at Port Kaituma, Guyana.

It was difficult to get into a school in January in the city of Georgetown, so I decided to go to evening classes to study for my GCSE classes. My parents could not afford for me to take five subjects at GCSE privately, but that's what was needed to start the registered nursing programme. As a result, I only took three subjects at that time which my family could afford.

My eldest brother was working in the police force during that time. He used to play cricket for the police force, and he was one of the fastest bowlers in the Guyanese police force. My brother took his salary for one month and paid for my exams. I remember he told me that God would support him that month and God did provide. I am so grateful to him and grateful to God for blessing him with the money, so he was able to give it to me.

My siblings and I are full of love. My mother taught us that love is of God because God is love.

One day I was walking down the street in the city of Georgetown and an elderly gentleman approached me. He said he was working at the Ministry of Health, and they were looking to recruit people who would like to do nursing.

The first thing that came to my mind was whether he was a magic man or something like that. How could he have known I wanted to be a nurse?

He went on to ask if I knew of anyone who was interested in becoming a nurse. He said if I knew of anyone, I should ask them to go to the Ministry of Health.

I asked him what the requirements were to enter the nursing school. He said five subjects at GCSE and four months in the Guyana National Service. I asked him if he had any proof that he was working at the Ministry of Health and he showed me his badge.

I mentioned to him that I only had three subjects at GCSE as I could not afford to pay for five subjects. He told me I could get into the practical nursing programme with three subjects to start nursing, then develop onwards to the registered nurse programme. He also told me that to do practical nursing, I had to take an aptitude test, then do national service for four months before starting the practical nursing programme.

I completed the aptitude test and completed five months of national service along with forty other nurses. The military course lasted five months instead of four months because the military plane which was transporting foodstuffs crashed causing the course to be delayed.

I was thankful to God that the military base was situated a few miles from Matthew's Ridge where I grew up. My family were still living there, so I was able to visit friends and get food as this was limited in the military camp due to the delay of food following the crash of the food plane.

My Pre-Nursing Military Experiences

Leaving the shores of Georgetown to venture out to the northwest region of Guyana was exciting. My only fear was thinking about the steamer having to travel through rough waters overnight for hours. Even though I was afraid, I knew I would see my family in Matthew's Ridge. I also thought that it was the beginning of a new life for me, as the orientation course for pre-nursing school was what I had dreamt of for years.

I had thoughts of turning back, but I remembered that the military experience was compulsory before I was able to get into nursing school. I mustered my faith, and I got on the steamer with the other nurses. It was a trip I knew so well. Our family used to travel on the steamer as flights were too luxurious in those times for the entire family to go on holiday.

There is a saying that people are less fearful when they know what to expect. As for me, I knew what to expect travelling on the steamer, but I was still fearful like a scaredy cat. The Atlantic waters are very rough, and the steamer used to toss to and fro. I've never forgotten those trips. Would I ever take those steamer trips again? The answer is no. I guess, only if my life depended on it.

This training course was productive, impressive and appreciated due to the high training content. We had jungle training and mock wars twice a week with loading machine guns. The mock wars were difficult, but they taught me survival. They taught me to be strong as a person in whatever I do. They taught me about self-discipline, resilience and determination.

We had to run a few miles every morning at around 5:30 a.m. before going onto the drill square. This meant waking up at around 5 a.m. and reaching the drill square at 5:30 a.m. ready for the day's exercises.

The self-loading rifle was difficult to run with for so many miles, but it taught me about self-discipline and reaching for my goals. It was another hectic task to do, but this taught me determination and perseverance.

The marching and weapons training took another hour of the morning, then it was time for the lovely breakfast. The peanut butter and bakes remain in my memory. To be honest, we did not have meal choices, so we settled for whatever was on the menu if it was not allergy related. It got worse after the food plane crashed.

MY PRE-NURSING MILITARY EXPERIENCES

I enjoyed the dismantling and assembling of the rifles. We had races to see who could dismantle and assemble their rifle the fastest. This helped me with speed when doing things.

The firing range exercise was once a week. It taught me about focusing. The bed-making lessons taught us how to make up a hospital bed. We were all skilful in bed-making when we left the military camp.

At times, the military camp experienced water shortages and the supervisors would share the limited amount of water. The mountain river was close by, but the captain instructed everyone not to go down by the river. He said if we went down to the river, we would not be able to continue the course. Only the regular staff had permission to go to the river.

If the captain had to stop anyone from completing the course, I believed that he would have had to stop all the nurses. This is because me and all the other nurses used to go down by the river where the water was flowing bountifully. No one wanted to use a small bowl of water when a river was within walking distance. The captain told us that using a small amount of water would teach us survival skills if we ever found ourselves stranded in the desert.

When it was almost time for the training course to be over, the plane that transported the food crashed. This delayed the course a little longer. The kitchen staff served the food in small parts as the storage room was running out of food.

Another nurse was also from Matthew's Ridge. We invited the nurses home to our families and collected whatever food we could get. We made sure we collected sugar and lemon and orange to make juice.

Myself and seven others did not go on the drill square on weekends, as we stayed in the camp dormitory and worshipped. The captain sent to ask us to go on the drill square during the second month. He realised that eight of us had not been going to the drill square for a month on weekends.

We decided to send back a message to say that we could not go to the drill square on weekends. The lance corporal returned and told us that the captain wanted to see us in his office. The lance corporal said that if we did not want to go on the drill square on weekends, the captain would have us sent back to the city.

Three of the nurses told me that they were dressing to go on the drill square. I told them I was not going to go to the drill square, but I would go to see the captain. They all decided to go with me.

When we reached the captain's office, he told us we were brave nurses. The captain took us to a spacious room and told us we could use that room every weekend to worship. We thanked him and stayed and worshipped for a while. The captain himself stayed with us for a while and sang songs.

We were grateful that the captain respected our religion and exempted us from the drill square on weekends.

Getting up every morning to run a few miles, then go on the drill square minutes afterwards was not easy but it was worth it. The captain asked us to go on the guard of honour parade which was a wonderful experience for me and the others. Thankfully, no one dropped their rifle.

My mother visited the military base when we had the guard of honour parade, as she was living at Matthew's Ridge. I was happy for her visit at the time of the parade.

Leaving the military base was sad, but I knew I had a dream to achieve.

Returning to the city after five months of strict intense training was a sigh of relief. I was still having aches and pains from the jungle wars and the miles of running every morning, but I was able to eat whatever I wanted and use as much water as I wanted. Overall, it was exceptionally good training, which helped to build me into a nurse with good discipline.

Returning to the city around May 1981, the wait for the nursing programme to begin took a while. When the course was completed, I did not look for a job in the city as I was waiting to enrol in the practical nursing programme. I spent a brief time in Matthew's Ridge where I took a small job at the post office.

My Practical Nurse Experiences

Finally, in October 1981 I began the licensed practical nursing programme, which was a two-year programme. I remember there were twelve of us who started the LPN two-year course. This was an incredibly special time for me. I told myself that my dreams were coming true. The other nurses seemed incredibly happy too. There were other nurses who started the registered nursing programme around that same time.

The beginning of the two-year programme seemed difficult for the first two months. The work included too many lessons packed together. I told myself that I could not back out, and I began to work and study harder. During the third month, the work began to get easier for me, because I started to focus more on the work. Everyone else was also doing well with the course.

The teamwork and team spirit in the group was amazing. We had effective communication with each other and we supported each other in terms of questions and answers. I remember we wore a buttermilk colour uniform for the licensed practical nurse programme. We did the practical aspect of our training in various wards and clinics.

When the two-year programme was complete, we were taught enough knowledge to equip our minds to complete the registered nurse programme.

It was a great experience for the group when we all were successful, and we graduated in November 1983. This was a happy celebration for every one of us. After working for two years post graduate, we could apply for the registered nurse programme. Most nurses from that batch eventually completed the registered nurse programme afterwards and fulfilled our dreams of becoming a nurse.

I worked at Georgetown Public Hospital following my LPN graduation. I also completed work experience out of district at Suddie Hospital which is in the Essequibo area. My elder sister Doris was living close to Suddie Hospital, so my out-of-town training experience was a good one. I had the privilege of working at the various health centres for six weeks of community experience. I got to know about all the various vaccines working at the health centres. I developed a good knowledge about children's clinics and antenatal clinics.

During my time working at Georgetown Hospital, I was in the nurses concert group and I was a part of the dance group. This was something that kept me happy, as most nurses were not happy due to overworking and small wages. Nevertheless, I was grateful that I had a job.

Dancing, both in Guyana and in England, always gives me confidence in my mind. Dancing is a form of exercise, and it also makes me feel good and gives me confidence in doing things. I am not a good singer, but I also used to sing in the nurses concert in Guyana. I presently sing in the choir group at church. I look forward to this every weekend. Singing is also another activity that builds self-confidence and practice makes perfect.

I remember the last nurses concert in Guyana. It was at the National Cultural Centre in Georgetown. Dancing and singing gives me joy. It makes me feel good about myself.

I still take part in concerts at my workplace, and I always choose dancing to do. I see it as an exercise and also as a way to build confidence. I may try yoga next.

My Life as a Midwife

My dreams were also to be a midwife and be able to deliver babies. I applied to go into the midwifery nursing school in 1986. I had to go out of town again for one year to collaborate with the midwives and get pre-knowledge experience before going into the midwifery school. I requested to complete the pre-knowledge training at a hospital in Matthew's Ridge as my family was living there and I grew up there. I also wanted to give back something to the place where I grew up. I was happy when the hospital matron sent me to work at Pakera Hospital in Matthew's Ridge. I spent a lovely and productive year working there. I knew the staff who were working at the hospital and this made it easier for me. As I was from Matthew's Ridge, I used to spend my days off at my mum's home. During working days, I mostly stayed at the nurses' hostel.

My trip back to the city after the one year was a smooth trip. I travelled by plane which was only a fifty-minute flight. I did not worry about the steamer, as the Ministry of Health paid my travelling expenses for the plane. Occasionally, I had the opportunity to take patients to the city. This was an opportunity for me to visit family and friends in the city after I had taken the patients to the hospital.

In May 1988, I gained entrance into the midwifery classroom at Georgetown Hospital. It was an exciting feeling for another dream to come true. I was successful with the out-of-town training programme. The midwifery course was also another challenging programme, but my heart and mind had one goal in sight. That was success. I focused and worked extremely hard, because I knew that a better life depended on me making the best out of my nursing career.

I loved the teachings of the delivery mechanism and I was astounded by the wonderful creative work of God. Learning the various stages of delivery, I was amazed.

Completing the midwifery programme made me understand more about God's beautiful creative work of pregnancy and delivery. It was a great feeling to see the newborn babies coming into this world. The cry of a newborn is heartwarming. What a wonderful God we serve.

I graduated as a midwife in 1990. The Gulf War was still in action. According to the news, the Gulf War sounded like it was war like a raging sea. It was awful. So many soldiers were losing their lives.

Nurses were on strike during that year for increased wages. I was amongst those nurses who were striking for increased pay. The hospital was mostly run by the army. The nurses and I did not want to leave the patients, but I believe at that time we were frustrated about overworking for little money and improper working conditions. Those days, nurses and assistant nurses did not have moving and handling equipment. Nurses used to physically lift patients. That is why so many nurses suffered with back issues.

My sister Jennifer went into labour to give birth to my niece Mellissa. I went to the hospital to see my sister. The ward sister told me that I had arrived at the right time to give a helping hand. The ward sister was happy to see me, as they were struggling with the amount of work.

I delivered my sister's daughter. My niece came flat out at birth with no cry. She was getting blue as she was not able to cry. I had to use all my delivery skills and thank God she began crying after massaging and suctioning to clear the airway. My niece jokes and says that I beat her at birth. Because it was my sister, I was worried at first, but I had to keep a brave face and go with the best action plan possible.

My sister asked how I was so brave and functioned as if nothing had happened. She told me that I did not scare her as I remained calm. When my niece was

MY JOURNEY AS A NURSE

well enough and everything was fine, I told my sister indeed I was scared but I could not have shown it.

My post graduate midwifery experience was very fruitful, very uplifting, motivating and inspiring.

After midwifery graduation, it was compulsory for each midwife to work at an out-of-town hospital for six months. I chose to go to Bartica Hospital. Bartica Hospital is a beautiful and small hospital. I enjoyed working there and had the privilege of collaborating with the amazing doctors, nurses and other staff there. My stay there at the nurses' hostel was only working on-call. The midwife only attended for deliveries. I do not think I can count the number of deliveries. Every day and night babies were born there.

Travelling from the city to Bartica with the steamer was not a problem. I was afraid of travelling with the speed boats. I used to travel home to the city when I had weekends off duty. Sometimes I had no choice but to use the speed boats when the steamer did not work.

I've always been afraid of the big rivers, as I do not know how to swim. Also, the speed boats were very noisy and made me feel sick.

I did not serve my full six months at Bartica Hospital as I had dreams of going abroad to work as a nurse. I decided to resign and make plans to travel abroad without securing a job overseas. That was like walking up the staircase in the dark without even seeing the next step. I call it faith in God according to my second book, *Unseen Steps to Victory*.

More than five of my nurse friends had already left Guyana after the nursing strike during the Gulf War. The government did not give us the increased wages we were looking for, so nurses left Guyana for better living abroad and better working conditions.

I did not know where my passage would come from or where I was going to stay abroad. My first thought was St. Lucia as I knew friends and family there.

The staff gave me a good farewell party at Bartica Hospital. I remember one of the doctors told me that I would make it anywhere because I was hard working. That was so touching to hear.

I returned to the city and told my elder sister Doris that I would like to go to St. Lucia.

She asked if I already had a job and I said no. She looked at me for a second, smiled and said, "If that is what you want, go for it."

The way she responded with such calm gave me the reassurance that she believed things could be possible.

St. Lucia Experience

I made preparations for my trip to St. Lucia, knowing that if I did not get a job, I would be back on Guyanese soil looking for one instead. This I did not want to happen, as my faith and belief told me everything was going to be fine. I kept faith and hope alive as I continued with my preparations to an unknown land. My family was not sure if I was doing the right thing, but just like me, they trusted in God that all would be well, and it was.

I left Guyana in April 1991. The Gulf War was ending around that time. This was my first trip out of Guyana. The flight to Barbados was smooth, as was the second flight from Barbados to St. Lucia. The airport in St. Lucia searched my bag asking if I had brought gold from Guyana. I told them I had my jewellery, but they were looking for raw gold.

When I reached St. Lucia, it was a whole unfamiliar environment for me with a different culture. It was difficult at first as I was getting to know the place and getting to know new people. It took me a while to get used to the broken French language. I love listening to it.

I visited the Ministry of Health in St. Lucia, and thankfully they were recruiting nurses from overseas. I met other Guyanese nurses in St. Lucia also.

I passed the nursing interview in St. Lucia and the staff at the Ministry of Health told me that as soon as they received my nursing transcript, I could start working.

St. Lucia's Ministry of Health was recruiting nurses at the same time, so God sent me there at the right time. My transcript was delayed in Guyana, so I waited for two months before I began working.

The Guyana nursing council was delayed with the transcript, but they finally had to release it. I remember it was $500 for the transcript in 1991. I would not want to imagine what nurses pay for that piece of paper now.

God was good to me during my two months waiting in St. Lucia, as I had enough money to keep myself afloat. I also had gold chains I bought in Guyana just in case my money ran out. I was able to sell the chains and the money kept me going.

Finally, I received the transcript, and I began working in another country away from Guyana. I had always dreamt of going abroad and it happened sooner than I expected.

ST. LUCIA EXPERIENCE

I worked at Victoria Hospital first from 1991 to 1998. I worked on medical and surgical units as well as the emergency unit and operating theatre. The time working at Victoria Hospital was mostly on the paediatric unit, so I had the privilege of dealing with babies and young children. I remember working on the paediatric unit when Hurricane Debbie passed. I thought that night would never end. Thank God it did. There were so many roadblocks from landslides. I did not get home until around 11 a.m.

Registered Nurse Accomplished Goal

The birth of my daughter in 1996 in St. Lucia reminded me and reassured me that nothing is impossible with God. In 1997, I bought a property in West Bank, Guyana as I was planning to go back to Guyana and live. I thought of going back to Guyana to complete the general registered nurse programme. I applied to go to the nursing school at the public hospital in Guyana, but there was no vacancy.

    I decided to contact the private nursing school at St. Joseph's Mercy Hospital in 1998. The director informed me that with my qualifications and experience abroad I could register, but I had to pay a hefty sum of money for the three-year nursing programme. I was happy with that as I was free to leave Guyana soon after the programme to return to St Lucia. My husband agreed eventually, and I resigned from Victoria Hospital in July 1998, and I began a three-year nursing programme in September 1998 at St. Joseph's Mercy Hospital in Georgetown, Guyana.

My daughter Crystal was just under two years old, but I took her with me to Guyana. I first stayed at the house I bought in the country area, but I was getting to classes too late. The floating bridge was closed off for long hours and I had to cross the river in a speed boat with my daughter to take her to my sister Doris. I then decided to rent out the house and use the money to rent an apartment closer to the nursing school in the city. It was a big apartment. The nurses used to visit sometimes after classes to study as a team.

My sister Doris used to babysit my daughter and take her to preschool. Life was easier as I did not have to worry about the floating bridge closing or the speed boat I was afraid of.

In 2001, I completed the three-year registered nurse programme. I remember the director called us from the classroom to show us the news. It was shocking to see. It was the 9/11 bombing and it was horrifying to watch.

The three years in the classroom and working on the units, theatres and clinics were challenging but God got us through those three years. The director was profoundly serious and every morning she would not start the class without telling us to pray and sing gospel songs. I still remember her saying to us, "Do not make all the money you paid go to waste. Pass the exams for yourself and your family. Walk out of here proud."

I was eager for the exam results to come out before my birthday on 3 November. I promised my family in St. Lucia that I was going to be back for my birthday.

The exams results were due in November and the results came out on 2 November. I thought I would not make it home for my birthday. The afternoon of 2 November, I called my sister Jennifer to give her the good news. On the other side of the phone, my sister did not welcome my message with joy, and I knew something was wrong. The same day my results came out, my mother had high blood pressure from the night before and no one said anything. Then my sister said my mother's blood pressure went up extremely high and she had a stroke. My celebration stopped that afternoon.

My big sister Doris organised a flight for me right away over the phone and the next morning I was on my way to St. Lucia on my birthday as I wanted but I was unhappy. I stopped over at Barbados for an hour and reached St. Lucia at 3 p.m. on my birthday. I asked the taxi driver to take me home to drop off my bag, then I went straight to the hospital. I spent the rest of my birthday with my mother at the hospital. The nurses knew me as I had worked there before.

My daughter was happy to see me as she went back to St. Lucia two months before me.

My mother never fully recovered from the stroke as she had to use a walking stick. Ten years later, she got sick with cancer. The doctor told my mum she had eighteen months to live. I visited St. Lucia when my mother was supposed to be having surgery for the cancer.

St. Lucia was expecting a hurricane, so all surgeries had to be cancelled and the hospital asked everyone to take their families home. Only the extremely ill patients stayed in the hospital. I took my mother home and one hour afterwards the hurricane began. It lasted from 2 p.m. and continued through the late hours of the evening. I remember my mother telling us to stay calm as the hurricane would be over soon. She was always a person with a strong faith in God. She has built my faith with so many things. My daughter and I had to go to the international airport by buying a plane ticket. The main road was damaged by the hurricane. I felt sad leaving my mother with the condition she was in.

She lived for two years after the diagnosis instead of eighteen months. She had complained of pain in her side, but the doctor told her it was muscle pain from the stroke without investigating it. Unfortunately, it was cancer. This doctor diagnosed it a while afterwards. She battled with cancer for two years. Her suffering is over now. She died on 12 March 2012. I had the privilege of seeing her and caring for her days before she died. I saw her take her last breath. She died at her home in Guyana. She requested to be looked after in Guyana where she was born. She chose to die in Guyana.

Tapion Hospital, St. Lucia

When I returned to St. Lucia in November 2001, during my post-nursing programme, I accepted a job at Tapion Hospital which is a private hospital. Sister John, who is a wonderful person, gave me the job. She was a very supportive sister to all the nurses. She did not regret her choice because I did my job well. To register in St. Lucia as a full registered nurse and midwife, I had to take the St. Lucia nurse exam at which I was successful.

Myself and two other nurses, Gail and Sonia, took the St. Lucia nurse exam at the same time. We passed the Guyana exams months prior in 2001. It was hard knowing that we had completed the nursing exams in Guyana and had to take another exam. To continue to work in St. Lucia, we had to complete St. Lucia state exams. We did not have to go back to nursing school. We only had to complete the exams. Thankfully, the three years of nursing school training were still fresh in our minds.

Myself and those two nurses Gail and Sonia returned to St. Joseph's Mercy Hospital in 2002 for the graduation. I can remember we travelled to Guyana on the same flight to attend our long-awaited graduation with excitement and a feeling of knowing we had made it. Nothing is impossible to those who believe.

I always said to the nurses that I believed the exam results would come out before my birthday and I would spend my birthday in St. Lucia. Due to my mum's stroke in St. Lucia the day before my exam results, I genuinely did not enjoy my success celebration. I travelled to St. Lucia on my birthday, 3 November 2001, the day after my exam results. I spent the rest of my birthday in the hospital at my mum's bedside. I was happy to see her alive nevertheless and she too was happy to see me. Celebration was nowhere in my mind for me and my family at that time.

Thankfully, my mum's condition stabilised and she made it, with a walking stick, to my graduation. It was like a bittersweet graduation.

It was lovely to catch up with everyone else from the programme at the graduation. We shared all the stories of classroom years which were different in months and years. There were happy days. There were sad days. There were challenging times and easy times. The nursing director was extremely strict, and she made us sing songs and pray before we began each class. Success was high on her list for us, so it was no time to muck around. I remember her saying,

"You need success not only for yourself but your family." She said, "Make yourself and your family proud," and indeed we did.

Sadly, our nursing school director passed on a year ago.

Special Miracles of Life

Every day is a miracle from God and God blesses us with multiple brand new mercies each new day. Nevertheless, sometimes things happen in our lives that we least expect.

When I migrated from Guyana to St. Lucia in April 1991, it was only a thought that came to my mind that I should seek a job overseas. I was not sure why that thought came to my mind. Looking back now, I know it was the plan of God. After that simple thought came to my mind about migrating overseas, two months later, I was St. Lucia bound. I did not know which country I wanted to go to at first, but I ended up choosing St. Lucia. Everything went well.

My sister Doris bought my first plane ticket out of Guyana. I was extremely excited to travel and make a better life for myself and my family.

I can remember around 1990, it was the Gulf War and nurses were on strike including myself. It was a grim time for the nurses in Guyana as the wages were not enough to pay the bills. The nurses were leaving the country despite the appalling transcript money.

The nurses' salaries remained dormant, despite the fact nurses were leaving Guyana in large numbers. I thought I had to make a move to get a better nursing life before I got older.

I can remember leaving the nurses' strike and going to the hospital to help deliver my sister Jenny's baby girl who is all grown up and has a pretty daughter of her own. I am so happy that back then I was already a midwife to help deliver my sister's baby.

Delivering babies was another way of seeing the miracles of God. I never counted the babies I delivered. There was no time to count.

I remember delivering babies at Georgetown Public Hospital, Bartica Hospital, Pakera Hospital, and Tapion Hospital. I remember sometimes on night duty I used to feel drowsy but when there was a delivery, all eyes had to remain open to ensure a safe delivery and to ensure that both baby and mother were doing well.

Hearing the babies' first cry and seeing their faces as they entered the world was an amazing thing for me.

Giving birth to my own daughter was another great miracle as the gynaecologist told me I may not be able to have children. Faith and hope were what I kept alive with prayer. Hope is like standing in the dark, looking out at the light. This is what I did for years.

Getting the opportunity to return to Guyana in 1998 to complete my registered nurse programme was another miracle for me.

The day one of my nurse friends gave me a contact number to call a recruitment team in England felt like a joke. First, I thought it was a prank, but I called the number. The next day I had an interview by telephone. One week afterwards I received my working visa. Two weeks after that my daughter and I caught our first flight to London. That was indeed another unexpected miracle from God. God does not come but he will send people to help us along the way. Climbing unseen steps is hope and faith together. This is profound and powerful.

I began working in England in 2005. It is now 2023 and I have never seen the person who recruited me. All I remember is that the person had an African accent, and I remember the person's name. He sent a taxi to collect my daughter and I from my aunt's home in Deptford to take us to Swindon. It was about an hour and a half to Swindon. We received a heartwarming welcome at Church View Care Home. The nurses' living apartments were just across the street from the care home. We spent about three years in Swindon before migrating to London in 2008. Church View Care Home was the first care home I worked at in England and Swindon is a beautiful small town.

The person who completed my interview was the owner for Hallmark Healthcare, one of the leading care home providers. I saw him sometimes when he visited Church View Care Home in Swindon. I enjoyed collaborating with that company too, but we migrated down to London in 2008 after my daughter was successful in an acting school audition. This was another miracle for the family as London is multicultural which is a good place for children to grow up and learn to associate with everyone from all walks of life. Swindon at that time was not diverse but it is getting better with this.

Becoming a registered care home manager was another miracle for me as I thought that all companies would have been unfair to me, but I was wrong.

American Experiences

As a child growing up, I always dreamt of going to America. People used to always talk about the Big Apple. People used to talk about Uncle Sam. People used to talk about the City of Light.

    My husband, my daughter and I first visited Brooklyn in New York City in 2004 for a two-week vacation. We stayed with my Aunt Melrose who is no longer with us. I remember my aunt took my daughter and I shopping in Brooklyn. Suddenly we heard gunshots and saw two youngsters running in our direction shooting at each other. My aunt told us to run for cover behind a parked car. This was like in the movies. It was so scary. When it was safe and all clear, we moved from behind the car. This was only two days into the vacation. On the fourth night, we heard bottles breaking on the ground floor of the building. People were fighting. My daughter and I decided that we would not return to New York City if that was how life was there.

    During our two-week vacation, one of my nurse friends Gail told me about her friends who needed a midwife to teach them how to care for their newborn.

It was a young couple and they were both teachers. I did not know them, but I took the chance to visit their home for the week they asked. I had to travel one hour by train. I spent about three days at their home teaching them everything about newborn babies. They were able to go out for one of the evenings while I babysat. At the end of my one-week teaching session, the couple gave me $1,000 and gifts. I can remember they both cried when I was leaving which made me emotional too. They were happy for the knowledge of newborn care. This was in 2004.

We returned a second time to New York City when my daughter was older. My daughter and I took a trip to Canada for four days and decided to pop across to New York with the coach for a day to see my aunt. This was our second visit to her. She had moved house, and we were so happy she did.

When we reached the coach station at Manhattan, we took the train to Brooklyn. There was this guy on the train who tried to form a conversation with us because he was from Guyana too, but I did not know him.

I told my daughter he seemed like he wanted to rob us, and I was right. When we got off the train, he was walking behind us. He said he would call his taxi driver friend. We told him we were waiting for someone just so he would leave. He was watching from a corner and saw we were checking for taxis and he returned saying his taxi driver friend was on the way. I told him we were fine, and he could leave. He was so persistent that I knew for sure he was up to something.

Finally, we got a city taxi and we got to my aunt's place safely. She called a family taxi to take us back to the coach station as we only spent the day with her. We were happy we did as she passed away two years afterwards with high blood pressure.

I visited my friend Pinkie in Huntsville, Alabama in 2019, and we made a visit to her brother Courtney in New York City. This was my third visit. The flight to New York that evening was very rough due to fierce winds and thick clouds. The plane circled the city about nine times before touching down in JFK. Once it was about to land, the winds blew the plane off the runway course and there was a sudden deep dive upwards. It was scary but God is good. Being on that plane felt like we were in the movies. I was afraid of flying back to Huntsville, but I did not have a choice. This visit was a wonderful one where we spent two days.

On the day of the flight back, we were kind to a taxi driver and let him take us to the airport as no one was taking him. His car was slow, and the traffic was busy. We missed the flight and had to buy new tickets to Nashville as there were no flights to Huntsville.

We flew back to Nashville just in time for dinner at the Cheesecake Factory restaurant with Pinkie's family. It was an excellent dining experience. After dinner, we drove down to Huntsville. The next day I flew back to London.

America is beautiful and England is beautiful. My choice of visiting America as a child has changed to a choice of England.

Climbing the Career Ladder

Life has a way of throwing obstacles in our pathway, but I have proven remarkable determination and perseverance in overcoming them. In the face of adversity, I have not only survived, but thrived. My ability to navigate through challenging times and appear stronger is a testament to my character. The challenges I met have shaped me into the incredible person I am today.

I have always known climbing to be a tricky thing. Workers who use a physical ladder for their daily job would recommend that you avoid looking down when you are climbing the ladder or even when you reach the top. Looking down the ladder sometimes makes people feel afraid of falling. Looking to the top of the career ladder may seem like a difficult task. Looking at people who have already made it to the top may seem like a hard piece of work.

The secret of success is taking your career one step at a time and that is what I did. I worked hard and kept my eyes on top of the ladder because I knew, one day, I would reach the top. I sometimes helped and supervised other nurses on my way upwards. My mother taught me that helping others is a way of also helping myself.

I started as an assistant nurse in 1981 and graduated in 1983. I completed the midwifery programme in 1988 and graduated in 1990. I completed the registered nurse programme in 1998 and graduated in 2002.

I became a care home trainer in 2005 at my first job in England after a series of trainers' courses in Wales, Bristol, Birmingham and London. These trainers' courses included dementia training, moving and handling training, food hygiene training and tissue viability training. As a trainer, I was able to help with staff training along with my manager job.

I worked hard as a deputy care home manager, followed by acting care home manager. Due to hard work and dedication, the boss promoted me to the registered care home manager seven years ago. It was not an easy task but with hard work and dedication to my job, I was able to conduct my dream of becoming a nurse and more.

I have learnt that to move from one destination to another, I have to move my feet. When I first worked at Church View Care Home, I accepted the opportunities to go on training sessions and trainers' courses. I accepted any training that came my way, and as a result I was able to help with training in the care home.

When my daughter completed her acting school audition, she was selected for the acting school in September 2008. We moved down to London for my daughter to start the acting school for two years. I used to take her every weekend to Piccadilly. It was £3,000 for the two-year course. It was a large amount of money those days, but I accepted it because we wanted to stay in London, as it is a multicultural place. This was the only way I was able to get the job transfer to London, which I did.

    I first worked at Ashmead Care Home without any issues because my qualifications were acceptable. Due to my trainers' certificates, I aided with training during my working time. This was a 110-room nursing home. Due to the expenses, I took a part-time nursing job one day a week at Sir Jules Care Home. The manager there asked me to aid with training and she taught me everything about the manager's job. The manager resigned months afterwards and opened her own business. From then on, the director gave me the role of acting manager. This was in 2010. Since then, I have been working in management.

A Black Person in the Nursing Arena

It was very difficult to get promotions according to my qualifications and experience in the past. Persistent excellent work with motivation and prayers helped me to get past this situation. It was very stressful sometimes, but I remembered that if I did not continue trying, I would not succeed.

I mentioned in my book introduction that you can only shoot an arrow by pulling it backwards. So, when life is dragging us back with difficulties, it means that it will launch us into something great. With prayer, trust in God and excellent work, I reached success. Through it all, I must say that I have pursued my career dreams and I thank God.

God created us all equal and we are all beautiful in the sight of God.

There are good people out there, but there will always be people who have hatred in their hearts for black people and other races. Sometimes even their own race. I had experiences of this, but I mostly experienced this years ago when it was time for me to get a promotion. My work was exceptionally good, yet as a black nurse, I had been detained for years from being promoted to a registered nurse manager.

I have been in my present company working as a registered manager for seven years. This helped me to understand that not everyone is unfair. I respect everyone for who they are, and where they come from. I would like people to show me that same respect.

There might be seldom times when I will have that strange look from someone from another race. That look of surprise. Sometimes people ask in a doubtful way, "Are you the manager?"

"Yes," I say with a lovely smile.

I, along with other black nurses, despite our high qualifications, struggled for years to be promoted. This situation seems to be improving a little due to equality and diversity policies.

A Prayer for Nurses and Healthcare Workers

> Give to my heart, oh Lord, compassion and understanding.
> Give to my ears the ability to listen.
> Give to my hands skill and tenderness.
> Give to my lips words of comfort and empathy.

Give to me, Lord, strength for selfless service and enable me to give hope to those I am called to serve.

Reaching Beyond My Career Dreams

It was a long difficult struggle that led me from success to success. It was nobody but God. He was the one who was leading me throughout all my difficulties. God was the one who was taking me up the rough side of every difficult mountain. God was the one who was taking me through all the dark valleys. It was not I, but the Lord.

My motto is never give up. Always aim for the moon. If you fall, you will land between the beautiful stars.

I grew up poor but contented and happy with dreams of being a registered nurse and midwife. God answered my prayers and from then to now he has taken me through struggles and smooth times, moving from step up to step up. There were times when I fell, but the good Lord picked me up. I was in the valley of decision, but God rescued me. My life is one trusted in God's will.

Now I am on top of the mountain, but I did not get there all alone. I thank God for making my dreams come true. I am now a registered nursing manager.

Leading a nursing care home with sixty-four rooms and sixty-five staff for eight years could be challenging, but God made my load lighter by blessing me with amazing staff, residents, relatives and an amazing multi-professional team. I know one hundred percent it is the hands of God and I give him all the praises and the glory.

I am so pleased that the chefs and the kitchen assistants were able to keep five stars every year for years. My staff and I passed the GSF with a platinum award.

Getting through six unannounced CQC inspections and hearing the inspectors saying, "Well done, there are no breeches. You have done very well," is an amazing feeling. Out of eight inspections, only two inspections needed minor improvements. My workplace has been overall "good" for years now. I am grateful to God and all my staff, the directors and the boss. We could not have done it without God. What an amazing God we serve.

The secret of success is putting God first and giving him thanks and praise every step of the way. The secret of success is helping to pull others up the ladder when you climb. Do that and God will give you extra strength on your way up the mountain.

The secret of success is giving even though you do not have much to give. I have been there. I gave my last and have been blessed double. We give not to get, but we give expecting God to bless us in return.

The secret of success is learning to dance in the rain until the storm is over.

Sometimes God leaves us speechless when his blessings come with overflow. That is the time we can share a bit more. The secret of success is releasing, letting go of your hurt and forgiving. The secret of success is loving your neighbours as yourself.

The secret of success is walking with God, speaking to him, praying and asking him to direct your path. The secret of success is trusting the will of God. The secret of success is building a better report on the action plans of failure.

The secret of success is seeing everyone equal to yourself because in God's eyes we are all created equal. Be proud of yourself and let us give all praises, thanks and glory to God.

Giving Up Is Not an Option

My motto is never give up. Always aim for the moon. If you fall, you will land between the beautiful stars.

I am a typical example of not giving up. I was a deputy manager, then acting manager for almost three years. When it was time to get a promotion, I was always passed over with silly excuses. I did not give up on wanting and trying to be a registered manager. I kept on trying until I succeeded in 2016.

People with weak hearts and weak minds give up easily, not knowing if they had pressed on a little longer, they would have experienced success. This happened to gold miners who gave up and other gold miners visited the same site and conducted remarkable success because of perseverance. Motivation, determination and perseverance are key to reaching remarkable success.

What our hearts and minds tell us, once we put it into action, we can achieve those goals.

I had discouraged hours and a few failures in life, but I took them as stepping stones to success. Just like me, you can use your discouraging hours and failures to set future goals. We learn from our mistakes and failures as these are great lessons to help promote us to higher grounds.

If your plan does not work, try another action plan which will lead you to your goals. It is the same as taking a taxi or a bus if the train workers are on strike. Try all means to get to your destination safely. In the same way, we should try hard to reach our goals with enormous success. I always worked hard and tried to do the best I could in every aspect of whatever I did. The beauty of success is being your best in whatever you do.

In failures, frustration and discouraging hours, say a prayer. Do something you like to do. Visit friends and family. Sing a song you like. Watch a funny movie. Try to think about people who have gone through worse times than you. These things will help you to understand that your situation could have been worse. Helping others who need your support will help you to motivate yourself. Sharing your experience with others will help you to release unhappy feelings towards your failures. Keep hope alive. Continue to think positively, knowing that there is always light at the end of the tunnel. Continue to look up and work hard towards your goals in life. Do not let anyone tell you that you cannot make it in life. With God in your life, nothing is impossible. Keep pressing on to your goals.

This is why I love to watch the Athletics Championships. Sometimes athletes are seconds away from winning the gold. I love when this happens. This tells us that sometimes we are just seconds away from reaching our fulfilled dreams that will give you the career arena you have been dreaming about. People may laugh at you and say that you cannot make it. This may get you down but continue to move on towards your goals in life.

I love victories. I love success. I love celebrations. I love getting to that stage of hearing "well done" and "congratulations". You are thinking the same. I use a brief word of prayer before I embark on any goal in life.

During the COVID-19 pandemic, I mentioned to my daughter Crystal that I would write my first book and get it publish in 2023. I can remember my daughter looked at me and smiled. She supported me as she told me she loved the inspirational messages I wrote on Facebook. That made me feel motivated. Then she said, "I know you will write a nice book, but I am not sure if people will buy your books as mostly celebrities and rich people are popular in book selling."

I laughed it off. I got a bit discouraged, but my daughter said, "But you can still draft your book as I am sure people will buy your books."

I told her I knew of people who wrote books but who were not rich or celebrities and they made it in the industry. My daughter Crystal said, "Ok, Mum, it is so true. Go for it."

In 2021/2022, I wrote my first book *Valley to the Mountain: Blessings and Lessons*. This book was published on 6 March 2023, and it is non-fiction.

In 2022/2023, I wrote my second book *Faith in God: Unseen Steps to Victory*. This book was published on 12 May 2023.

From January to April 2023, I wrote my third book on weekends and nights called *Professional Excellence: Education Is the Key*. This book was published on 6 November 2023.

This is my fourth book, *My Journey as a Nurse*. I am not perfect, and no one is but God. If I can write four books and I do not have a broad experience in writing books, then you too can reach anything you want to do once you put your heart, your soul and your mind into it.

God did not promise us a smooth life all the time, but he promised to be there to protect us and guide us through. The same with the roads you drive on. There are smooth roads and bumpy roads. When you reach the bumpy spots on the roads, you drive slowly and carefully. Your car will break down sometimes, but you do not leave it on the road. You get it fixed. It is the same with going for your goals. When we fall, we do not stay down. We must get up, brush off and keep going. The race is not always for the swift but for all those who endure to the end.

In the recent World Athletics Championships, I saw someone was coming first in the race. She fell three seconds before the finish line and the person who was coming second touched the finish line first. Oh yes, these things happen often. Stay on course. Keep looking at the finish line. Focus on the finish line. Do not look at what anyone else is doing. Focus on your dream goal or goals. I love the saying "going for gold" and I also love the part of achieving "gold". We all do. For ourselves, our families and friends. Dreams were meant to be conducted by the dreamer. Let your dreams become reality. Please never give up as I always say giving up should not be an option. Keep on going to the finish line to reach your goals.

Once someone graduates, it means that they did not give up on their studies. If that person gave up on their studies, it would mean they would not be able to graduate.

Going through schools, colleges, universities and other academic institutions is a very difficult process. The goal is to aim for success with hard work and dedication. The end results will be a happy one.

Congratulations to My Daughter on Her Great Achievements

Thanks to my daughter Crystal Johnson who has made me proud with her hard work and dedication She completed her English degree in 2018 at Queen Mary University of London and her master's in law 2022 at the University of Law, London. Congratulations again to her. This was not easy, but with the help of God, Crystal made it through the hard work.

Graduation of Three Family Members on the Same Day: 11 November 2023

Graduations are great, happy and priceless moments that will be memorable forever. What an impressive God we serve. God is still the greatest.

My nephew Dameion Mark McLennon completed a Commonwealth master's of public administration. It was about three years ago and he graduated from university also.

This was a difficult couple of years for Dameion, but he has worked hard for what he wanted. You have braved it through the storms. Dameion always says to me that God is the greatest.

My niece Yvonne Nikita Shelto Halley completed her bachelor's in public management. It was a double celebration for her because 11 November is also her birthday. She got married in August 2023 which was less than three months before her graduation. The two special celebrations in one year were priceless. Yvonne had issues with her laptop shutting down often and her work disappearing but her faith in the struggles granted her success.

My cousin David graduated as a doctor on the same day with my niece and my nephew. They were all in the same building graduating together. Congratulations again to them all.

My cousin Dr David has great faith with the hard studies over the years. She was not about to give up, so she pressed on and now she has reached her goal.

I chose to share these graduation stories under this chapter about not giving up. I knew of the difficulties these family members went through to accomplish success.

I went through difficult times as well to attain success. This is why I share these stories because I know that there are nurses, also care workers, who are out there struggling and want to give up.

I recommend that you focus on your dreams. Keep your eyes on the goal. Stay focused and set your priorities straight. Work hard. Pray and endure your struggle. Stay on course and go and claim your success. Nothing good comes easy. You can do it.

My Management Work Life

The yearly workplace barbecue usually takes place in the big gardens at work as the invites were usually in large numbers. This was a special occasion that myself, the staff, the residents, their families and the professionals looked forward to every year. This was another occasion not only for socialising and improving happiness and well-being for everyone, but also for bonding and enhancing a greater professional relationship with the staff, families and visiting professionals.

During the COVID-19 pandemic we missed the barbecue so much, but we had to not only shield ourselves and others but follow strict government guidelines which were vital to save lives. Social gatherings were restricted during the pandemic, so we could have only dreamt about the barbecue.

During August 2022, we were able to socialise in the garden for our yearly barbecue. It was a beautiful day with lot of delicious food and a lot of visiting friends, families and professionals. The day was warm, and the sun was barely shining. The rain clouds were moving away and returning often but thankfully it did not rain.

Unfortunately, for the 2023 barbecue, we had to hold it indoors. The weather for August for the date we chose was showing a warm sunny day. The weather dramatically changed to a rainy day. Typical British weather. It is unpredictable. One cannot always be one hundred percent sure about British weather. Nevertheless, the barbecue went on very well indoors. We had an enjoyable time. It was like if no one realised it was an inside barbecue as everyone had a lovely time. It was my last barbecue at my workplace unless I visit for future barbecues.

The pandemic of COVID-19 has taught me how serious and how vital it is to find enough time for family and friends including finding time for myself. The pandemic also made me realise how precious life is as people were dying every day by the thousands all over the world. It was a time when I was able to reflect on my life and realise that I needed to give enough time for myself.

I remember during the pandemic nurses and carers were off sick. Doctors were off sick. It was a time that seemed like it would never end. It was like being on a boat in the raging sea. I had nurses who left the workplace as they were not allowed to work at two workplaces during the pandemic as this was against the policy due to potential risks of cross contamination. Five nurses left because of this.

During this same time, three other nurses fell sick to this killer virus. Carers also fell sick. It was a time when the isolation phase was fourteen days. We survived and made it through by the grace and mercies of Almighty God. I can remember my deputy manager and I used to go in on night duties to give the medication and to help the carers. During the day we were both on the unit as nurses were off sick. Not sure how we survived but God was in control, and he still is.

I remember looking after residents who had COVID-19. I was scared but I did not have a choice as someone had to care for those who were sick.

It took over a year before I contracted the virus which was in February 2021. The pandemic began in 2020. Thankfully, the nurses and carers were back to work when I went off on my fourteen-day isolation period. Luckily, my daughter did not catch the virus from me because both of us practised effective infection control measures.

Unfortunately, later in 2022, my daughter got the virus early in the year and again in June 2022. She was sick but she was still able to move around and do things for herself, for which we give God thanks. Some of the people were bedbound, and millions did not make it through the pandemic.

I thought the pandemic would never end but thank God it finally did. I never wanted to take the COVID-19 vaccine, but it was needed to stay in the job. It was emotionally disturbing to have to be forced to have something injected into my body against my will. It was dreadful and appalling but I am thankful I did not get sick with the vaccines like others who assumingly died from them.

My daughter Crystal and I travelled to the Caribbean in June 2022 for a family and friends' reunion in St. Lucia and Guyana. It was a happy reunion to see family and friends after the pandemic who we believed we might not have been able to see again. It was a God blessed privilege to see family and friends again. The vaccine cards came in useful because St. Lucia wanted the vaccine cards on entry.

We had a wonderful time in both St. Lucia and Guyana with family and friends. We had reunion dinners in both countries. They were beautiful and priceless occasions.

On returning to the UK in July 2022, I realised that I had to give up my five days a week nurse manager job and find more time for myself and my family. Pandemic and sickness are things that make people realise that family and friends are more precious than money, diamonds or gold. I remember during the pandemic people were talking about family and friends and there was no talk about money. This says a great deal about how inferior money is when family is needed.

On 18 September 2023, I thought long and hard and came to the final decision that I needed to give up my five days a week nurse manager job. It was a battle to decide to leave a job I loved so much for so many years. Nevertheless, there comes a time when we need to put ourselves and our health and happiness before our career, money and so much more. After careful thoughts and praying about it, I made up my mind to resign and this was what I did on 18 September 2023.

I was just getting a bit tired of the five days a week job and the fact that I was on-call twenty-four-seven as a manager did not make it easier. If a nurse called off sick and no agency nurses were available, as a manager I had to fill in the gap. I was not getting enough substantial time for myself and my family. Having to do the night checks and leaving my home at night if no night nurse was available was exceedingly difficult.

There is a time and a season for everything. Now I have resigned from my manager job, I believe in my heart it was the right thing for me to do at the age of sixty-two after forty-two years in the nursing arena. I wanted to resign with immediate effect, but my boss reminded me that I needed to give three months' notice. I laughed and said I would. He is the best boss I have ever worked with. He is kind, humble and a nice person. I will miss everyone at my workplace, and I am grateful and thankful to everyone there for their support and cooperation.

My three months for my resignation was supposed to end on 18 December 2023 but my boss asked me if I could work until the end of the year which I agreed.

I have been collaborating with the company for eight years. An amazing company with good CQC inspection ratings.

Cultural Day Concert at Work

This type of event is something that we hosted every year at my place of work. This is a special event that brings the staff, residents, families, friends and the professionals together. I love this time of the year when the cultural concert comes around, as it gave me a chance to do something for the residents, the staff and others who attended our yearly concerts. I enjoyed reciting poems, singing and dancing. I loved the dancing with the other staff. The residents enjoyed these concerts very much. I loved to see the smiles on their faces. Occasionally, the residents would sing along to the songs. These were precious moments to see residents singing along and residents sometimes danced along with us when we completed the various dancing. This is something I organised every year and everyone used to look forward to the yearly cultural celebration.

The community nurses occasionally would read a poem or give a speech. The staff were always given the opportunity to wear clothes from their cultural backgrounds. The staff chose to wear their usual uniform, which was their choice, and I respected their choice. The kitchen chefs usually prepared a choice of cultural dishes for the concert, and everyone usually enjoyed these delicious foods.

Birthday Celebrations

I love birthday celebrations. Every year I buy a special lunch for all my staff from the catering service for my birthday. I use my own money to do this. Apart from my birthday, I buy lunch for the staff sometimes. The staff do not like their birthdays to be made known, so I give them little gifts.

Every Christmas, I usually buy a small gift for every staff member from my own money apart from the Christmas voucher they receive from the company.

I once bought seventy-two small "well done, thank you" trophies for the staff. Sometimes my staff would say to me that I will spend all my money. I usually smile because I have learnt over the years about effective management skills. Showing gratitude to my staff with small tokens of appreciation and often buying them little treats has encouraged and motivated them to keep doing their best. It is a way of saying thanks to my staff for their support and cooperation and for the demanding work they are doing.

I love to give little treats now and then to show my gratitude and appreciation for the challenging work they are doing and continue to do.

On 3 November 2023, I held my special birthday lunch at my workplace for the last time as I would not be working at my workplace anymore in the new year. This birthday lunch was incredibly special. The night staff surprised me at my birthday lunch with a beautiful bunch of flowers, a heartwarming card and a gift voucher card just to say happy birthday and thanks for the support throughout the eight years collaborating with them.

Bonfire Night

As a nurse manager, fireworks on Bonfire Night are something that my staff and I, along with the residents and families, look forward to every year. We usually have this celebration around the end of October to the first week in November. We will choose an evening around 5:30 p.m. as it is usually dark already at that time in winter.

We often give glowsticks to the residents while they sit and watch the fireworks. The nurses and carers share the drinks and fingers foods, sandwiches, and other little snacks of preference. The staff will take photos of the fireworks and send them to staff who were unable to attend the occasion. People feel a little disappointed when all the fireworks are finished as it was lovely to sit and watch the beautiful sparks.

Lights are always something that I love to see, especially the Christmas lights.

The fireworks always bring smiles to everyone faces.

Unannounced CQC Inspections

I worked as a nurse manager in care homes for thirteen years. I worked as a deputy manager, I worked as an acting care home manager, but I worked as a registered care home nurse manager for seven years until now.

Throughout those thirteen years of management experience, I attended about ten CQC inspections. Out of the ten inspections, only one inspection I consider announced. This was when an inspector called the care home and I answered the phone. She said she was two minutes away from my workplace trying to find the place. I directed the inspector, and the inspector was there in less than a minute. She told me she was coming to do the inspection when she was a minute away. It was announced, yet unannounced. Not sure what others would say it was.

Out of the ten CQC inspections I attended at places I worked at in a managerial role, only two inspections needed required improvements in certain areas of the five key elements of inspection.

Getting through eight inspections I thank God for granting me the knowledge and wisdom with my management experience. I thank God also for always giving me skilled staff who are supportive, hardworking and knowledgeable.

It takes a good team with good teamwork and a team spirit. Passing the inspection with the COVID-19 health inspector was also a valuable experience for my staff and I.

The kitchen staying at five stars throughout my eight years at my workplace is also amazing. We still have our five-star rating in the kitchen and the overall workplace stays with a good rating. I am grateful and thankful first to God, then my staff, directors, the visiting professionals and the boss of the company, as everyone played a role in making the workplace so successful.

On 14 November 2023, the receptionist came to my office and told me that there were two people standing in the car park and they looked like CQC inspectors. She said that they had on badges. I told her that they were inspectors, and she should go back to the reception to open the door when they arrived.

They stood in the car park for a minute or two before pressing the doorbell. When they arrived at reception, they asked to see the manager, Lynette Johnson.

I at once went to the reception area and introduced myself, as my office is close to the reception area. I recognised one of the inspectors who was at the previous inspection.

It was only a one-day inspection and thank God it went very well and the inspection feedback at the end of the day was good. The leading inspector asked me to convey his thanks to the staff for a job well done. The service manager was in, and we were both pleased with the inspection.

I welcomed this inspection a great deal as it tied into the time when I had resigned from my work to leave at the end of the year by God's will.

After going through ten inspections, this has made me an exceptionally good manager. I did not add the yearly kitchen inspections because the chefs are great with managing the kitchen inspection. Inspectors showed up when we least expected them. It is the same as our blessings. Sometimes blessings show up when we least expect them. This is why any workplace should always continue to do the correct thing which is right.

15 November 2023

I held a general staff meeting to say thanks to the staff and to convey feedback on the inspection. I also bought pizza and chicken treats to say thanks. One of the kitchen staff had her birthday so she brought cakes, sweets and juice too. This all blended nicely together. Along with the happy birthday song, it was a thank you to all staff.

With our planned Christmas party on 14 December 2023 and my last day at my workplace on 29 December 2023, by God's grace, I am sure I can look back and be well pleased with my accomplished goals.

The future is in God's hand, but I pray that the new year will take me into the new pastures I prayed for. I had years of five-day work weeks and being on-call twenty-four-seven.

It is time for a change in my life, as sometimes we all need to take a step backwards and think about ourselves. At my age of sixty-two, I would like to be working less than five days a week.

I previously did care home training, so I might do training for the new year, which is another of my favourite jobs. I am a dementia trainer, a moving and handling trainer, and a food hygiene trainer. At least I will be able to do something I like and also for less hours. I would not have to be on-call twenty-four-seven, which will be good.

I will be able to spend more time on writing books which is one of my hobbies. This will also give me more time to spend with my family.

Summary

Life has a way of throwing obstacles in our pathway, but I have shown remarkable determination and perseverance in overcoming them. In the face of adversity, I have not only survived, but thrived. My ability to navigate through challenging times and to appear stronger is a testament to my character.

The challenges I met in my nursing career have shaped me into the incredible person I am today. My advice to all nurses and those who are dreaming of becoming a nurse is not to give up on your dreams. Giving up should never be an option. You may never know what lies ahead on the green grass if you do not take the first step. Failing to prepare is preparing to fail. Take the first leap of faith and trust God to take you to the other step. I took a leap of faith trusting God to grant me my dream goals, but God has granted me more than I dreamt of.

Each new morning God grants us new grace and mercies, but sometimes extra miracles happen when we least expect them. I can testify to this on occasions that God is good.

This advice about not giving up is not only for nurses but for anyone who believes that giving up is the answer because it is not the answer.

Nursing is a rewarding and fulfilling job, especially when patients recover. This is an extraordinary joy when this happens. I must confess, it is not the easiest of jobs, but difficult like most jobs. To make nursing look easy, one needs to love the nursing job, to do it well and do it from one's heart holistically and effectively.

Forty-two years of nursing, midwifery, care home training and care home managing has given me wonderful experience and knowledge I never imagined I could have. I have written three books, and this is my fourth.

My books entail stories mostly about myself and family. The years of knowledge and experience have given me a great insight into life and so many things to write about.

My journey as a nurse began forty-three years ago and it was an amazing dream that came true for me. Hard work and dedication were what I needed to climb the ladder of success in the nursing arena. There were days of struggle and difficulty where I was not sure if it was possible to move up the mountain, but nothing is impossible once we believe that we can do it with the help of God.

SUMMARY

I prepared for success. I did not prepare to fail. I set my mind to the things I wanted to achieve, and I went for what I wanted to achieve with all my willpower. I prayed and put God first in everything and success followed.

It does not matter where you are now. It is setting your mind for where you would like to be. This was always my motto. I started my first book during the pandemic and here I am on my fourth book. Determination, perseverance and resilience along with hard work pays off. If you take time to read my four books, you will understand what I went through, yet I did not give up.

I started writing around 2010, and I have been sharing my stories and inspiring messages on various social media platforms. I opened a social media page called the Message of the Cross. I have only shared inspirational quotes on this page, along with faith and miracle stories.

On the other social media platforms, I share inspiring daily messages, photos and uplifting songs. I love to write anything that may be useful for people going through rough times or those who may welcome such encouraging words.

My journey as a nurse was strongly dependent on the spiritual side of my life, which is prayers and trusting God for success. Nursing is a profession needing resilience, faith, courage and hope. Hope, as I mentioned previously in my book, is the feeling of being in the dark and looking out to the light. The only way we can reach the light is by prayers, trust in God, hard work and dedication.

Nurses, I recommend that you all believe in yourself. That was what I did. Tell yourself you are going to make it. Keep looking at your career goals and aspirations. Keep climbing the ladder of success. Only look down if you would like to help someone with their climb. I always believe that when we help others, it is another way of helping ourselves.

According to Florence Nightingale, who we knew as the nurse with the lamp, she too believed in the higher power who is God. She believed that there is a spiritual divine side of nursing. In her pledge for nurses, Florence Nightingale mentioned God. She was known for her care with professional excellence. This noble lady worked her way through the night with a lamp caring for the soldiers.

I had the privilege of collaborating with nurses in Guyana, St. Lucia and England, who showed such good qualities as Florence Nightingale. I read a great deal about her, and I practised excellent quality nursing throughout the forty-two years I have been working in the medical arena.

SUMMARY

Tips on My Next Book

This will be a small book of inspirational quotes. I am already halfway through this book, as writing is one of my hobbies. I have decided to make it into a small book, because it will be easy and handy to take around with you.

Please do keep a look out for this book, which I guess should be published around the end of February or March 2024.

This small book of inspirational quotes will not only inspire nurses but it will inspire anyone who reads it. It is a motivating, uplifting and inspiring book.

Reasons for Sharing My Stories

To inspire and motivate young nurses and nurses-to-be not to give up on their dreams. Especially those who have dreams of becoming a nurse one day.

To motivate anyone who is aching from one thing or another and feels that they cannot go on.

To remind all nurses that they are special, and they are doing a special and demanding job.

To remind all nurses not to accept disrespect from anyone whatsoever. Demand respect at all times. I always stand up for my nurses and carers when they are being disrespected by anyone.

To remind people that dreams were meant to be achieved.

To remind readers that failure does not mean that goals cannot be achieved. Failures are lessons and stepping stones to success.

To inspire nurses who are stressed out. I know, just like I struggled during my nursing career, other young nurses may be going through similar situations. If I can get through those challenging times, any nurse can. You just need that faith and resilience, and you will make it. Not only nurses, but anyone can overcome the hurdles of life once they set their mind to do so. Please do remember that no condition is permanent. There are always changes. Pray, trust God, work hard and keep a focused and positive mind.

To let people know that it is never too late to become a nurse. Just like any other job, you still have a chance at twenty-five years old. You still have a chance at thirty years old and over.

With the unprecedented and uncertain times, nurses as well as other people are getting frustrated with the cost of living and so much more. Reading my book will help them be able to believe in themselves and keep hoping and trusting God that things will get better for them.

Acknowledgments

The good Lord, my families, friends and mentors were there along the way to give me the necessary support and guidance I needed.

Thanks to my daughter Crystal who has always been supportive and encouraging. When I feel discouraged, Crystal always says encouraging words to motivate me. And I do the same for her. She always complies to the law books as she is legally strict.

During her studies at the various universities, I verbally motivated her, but I did not have to help her with her assignments or anything like that. She was exceptionally good and quick with her assignments. I am thankful and grateful to God for having her.

She has made me proud with her hard work and dedication. She has completed her English degree and her master's in law. Congratulations again to her.

Special thanks to my amazing publishing firm of Patrick and his team. I am so thankful and grateful for all the exceptional work everyone has done with my earlier three books. I have no doubt that you will do a fantastic job with this fourth book. Thanks a million to you all. Thanks to all of you for your excellent customer skills, communication skills, great feedback, professional work and for always delivering excellent job satisfaction. Well done, everyone.

Thanks to everyone who I have worked with in the various hospitals, health clinics and care homes, including my present workplace. This includes the doctors, nurses, all the other staff and supervisors, nursing school tutors and the directors and other professionals.

Special thanks to Nurse Rita Ramdayal, who is no longer with us. She was a great amazing nursing teacher. She taught us that we should never start a classroom day without singing songs of praise to God and pray. I will never forget the speech she gave us every week during the three-year training programme. Nurse Ramdayal told us that we should not let the money we paid for the training go in vain. She went on to say that if we do not prepare, then we should prepare to fail. She told us that we should walk out of the nursing school as proud nurses with our heads high and shoulders square. What was touching was when she said that we were not doing it for ourselves only. We were also doing it for our families. It hit home that families were depending on us to do well and not only for ourselves. I remember the daily song we used to sing. It was "Victory, Victory Shall Be Mine". Indeed,

ACKNOWLEDGMENTS

we all walked away from the classroom victorious. Glory be to God.

Special thanks to my boss and CEO, Amar, who gave me my first registered nurse care home manager job in England in 2016. He respected me for who I was and where I came from. He respected my high qualifications and treated the outcome of my interview with high respect.

I started in the company in 2015 as a deputy care home manager. With persistent hard work and dedication to my job, I was promoted to acting care home manager in the same year. My hard work continued and later, I was promoted to a registered care home manager in 2016 on my birthday. They were indeed happy and priceless moments. I was grateful and thankful.

This company has exceptionally good ratings with CQC inspections. There were challenging times, but the good times outweighed the tough times. I love my job. It was great news three days ago on 14 November 2023 when my workplace had an unannounced inspection by two CQC inspectors. It was reassuring to hear at the end of the inspection that it was a particularly good inspection. The leading inspector told me and the visiting service manager thanks. He also asked me to convey thanks to my staff for a job well done. I am thankful to the CQC inspectors for the way they conducted the inspection with great professional excellence.

Thanks too to my amazing and diligent staff. Thanks to my workplace service manager Shelley who has been working tirelessly to support the home to ensure that my staff and I adhere to all the compliances of the workplace.

Working together with good teamwork and good team spirit was what made the work lighter. There were minor conflicts at times amongst staff, but these were sorted at once due to my excellent management skills and my special management style.

I am grateful and thankful to my staff because they were also supportive towards the smooth running of the care home. Not only because of the little tokens of appreciation but because they are genuinely skilled staff. They were always supportive not only with work but also with the social activities of the care home such as barbecues, concerts, birthday get-togethers and so much more. They are special and gifted in their own ways.

Special thanks to my sisters Doris and Jenny who helped babysit my daughter Crystal when she was a baby to the time we migrated to England.

Special thanks also to my two nieces who also played a role in babysitting my daughter despite they themselves being still underage. They used to help their mum with the babysitting duties. With all

ACKNOWLEDGMENTS

the babysitting help I was getting from families, this allowed me to be able to complete my nursing programme and nursing duties.

Looking back now it makes me realise how time flies. My daughter is all grown up. Crystal completed her English degree at Queen Mary University in 2018. She went on to law school and graduated with a master's in law.

My nieces Mellissa and Tisha who used to help babysit Crystal, they too are all grown up. As the saying goes, time waits on no one. How time flies.

Special thanks also to my mum who also contributed with babysitting my daughter when she was a baby. Sadly, Mum passed on 12 March 2012. My mum and dad are no longer with us, but they were incredibly supportive of me to further my nursing career. My mum and dad were both alive when I completed my nursing programme. I will forever be grateful to them for the great values they instilled in me and my siblings. I remember my father words. He said, "I told you that you were going to be a nurse." I got my heart's desires, and my family too was also happy. Completing my nursing studies was especially important to me in so many ways. It was worth it to an exceedingly high extent.

I can remember when I got my first nursing job in St. Lucia and my mum paid $500 for my transcript. In 1991, that was a great deal of money for ordinary people to get. My mum was happy to help, and she had no regrets. I miss her and my dad dearly, but they have done well with their earthly chores. May their beautiful souls continue to rest in peace.

Special thanks to everyone who taught us in the Guyana National Service during our nurse orientation course. This course prepared us for the nursing career journey. This training course taught me so much about survival. It taught me that despite inconvenient situations, I must never give up. It taught me about resilience, perseverance and motivation. It was a very inspiring course.

Special thanks to my husband Walter Johnson who supported me financially throughout my nurse training. I remember when I wanted to return to Guyana for the three-year programme, he was not in agreement, but he eventually settled for the idea. He knew I was determined to reach my goal of becoming a registered nurse.

Special thanks to the staff at Tapion Hospital who were incredibly supportive and gave me a great send off to England. It was me and another nurse Gail who had our farewell party together. We left St. Lucia around the same time in 2005.

Special thanks to my dear friend Gail who gave me the phone number for the recruiting nurse agency in England. First, I thought it was a joke as sometimes she used to make little jokes and had us laughing at

ACKNOWLEDGMENTS

work. Well, that time she was serious because someone answered on the other end of the telephone line in England. I had my telephone interview and documents were sent to me within a week. Three weeks afterwards, my daughter and I were on our way to London for the first time. My Aunt Patsy welcomed us at Gatwick Airport. She was happy and excited to see us. So, with a little kindness from my friend Gail in giving me a phone number by God's will in 2005, my life, my husband's life and my daughter's life changed for the better.

God works in mysterious ways and I am grateful and thankful to him the most.

My dreams have been accomplished beyond measure.

Glory be to God.

www.ingramcontent.com/pod-product-compliance
Lightning Source LLC
Chambersburg PA
CBHW071400080526
44587CB00017B/3141